The Pig of Happiness

for Sarah

HarperCollins*Entertainment*
An Imprint of HarperCollins*Publishers*
77–85 Fulham Palace Road,
Hammersmith, London W6 8JB

www.harpercollins.co.uk

Published by HarperCollins*Entertainment* 2004
1 3 5 7 9 8 6 4 2

Copyright © Giles Andreae

The Author asserts the moral right to
be identified as the author of this work

A catalogue record for this book
is available from the British Library

ISBN 0 00 716097 6

Printed by Proost

THE PIG
OF HAPPINESS

There was once
a PIG

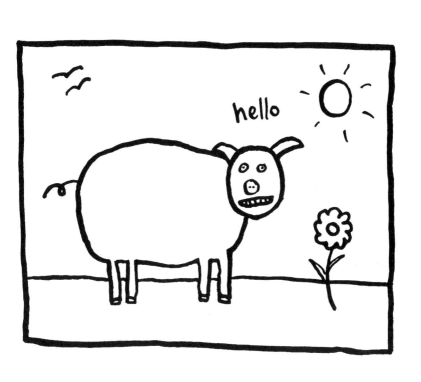

He was an ORDINARY
PIG in all ways

But one thing did
SET him APART

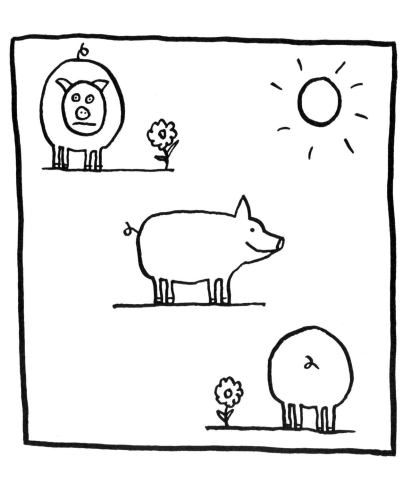

This thing was his DISTASTE for the MUMBLING and GRUMBLING that is the Natural Way with pigs

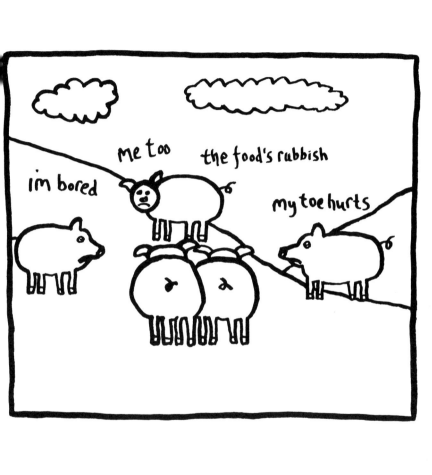

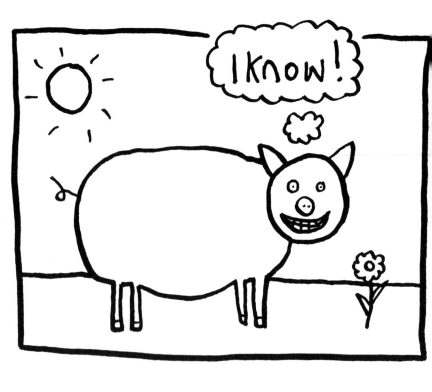

... thought the PIG

I shall become an

EXTRAORDINARY

PIG !

From now on I shall
stand for everything
that is

LIGHT

and

BEAUTIFUL

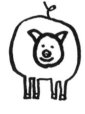

and TRUE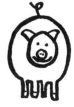

and

WONDERFUL

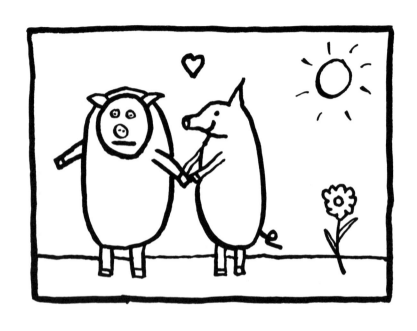

I shall see the BEST
in EVERYONE

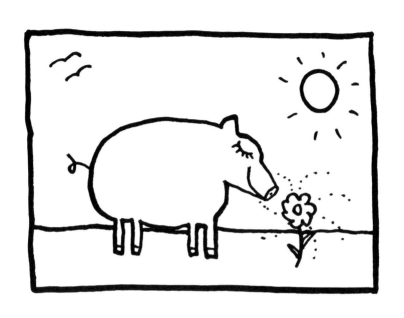

and the BEST
in EVERYTHING

I shall become ...

...THE PIG
of HAPPINESS!

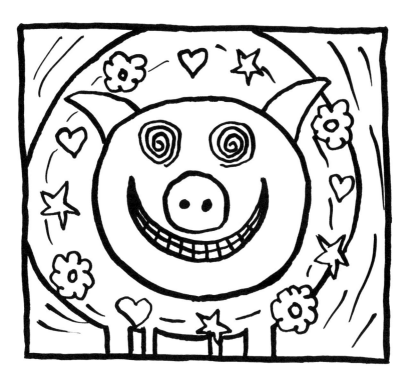

and so it did come to pass

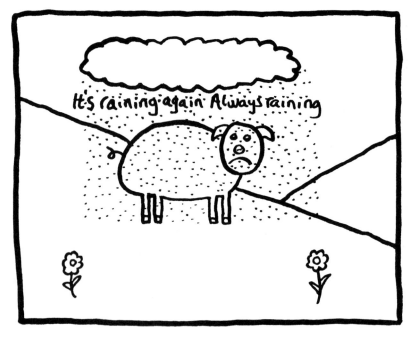

The next day, when Pig A COMPLAINED about the weather...

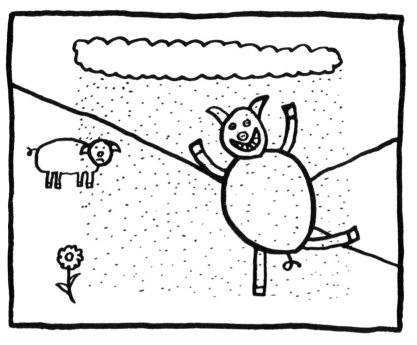

The Pig of Happiness went
DANCING in the rain

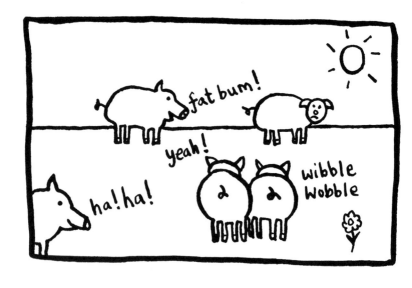

The day after that, when
Pig B was RUDE about
Pig C's bottom and all the
other pigs joined in...

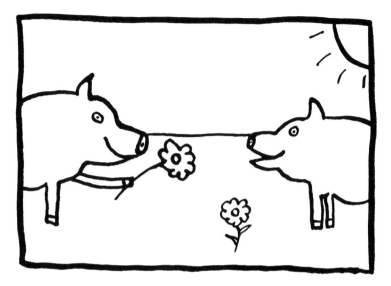

The Pig of Happiness gave
Pig C a FLOWER and
said in front of all the other
pigs that he thought Pig C
had a BEAUTIFUL bottom
actually

And so it continued daily

After a while, the Pig of
Happiness became so HAPPY
with being happy that his
HAPPINESS became too
BIG

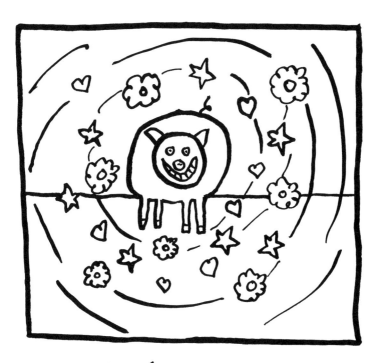

It had to find an ESCAPE

And so it was that it began to LEAK and SEEP from inside him into all the OTHER pigs

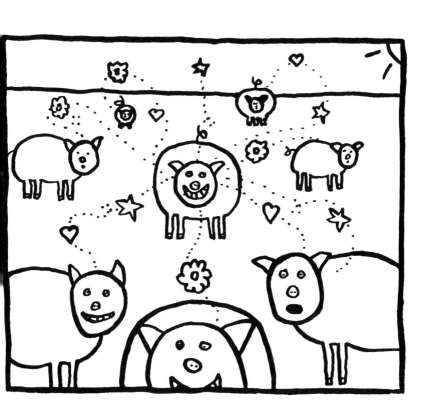

Now ALL the pigs are
HAPPY

And their HAPPINESS
is beginning to show signs
of LEAKING too

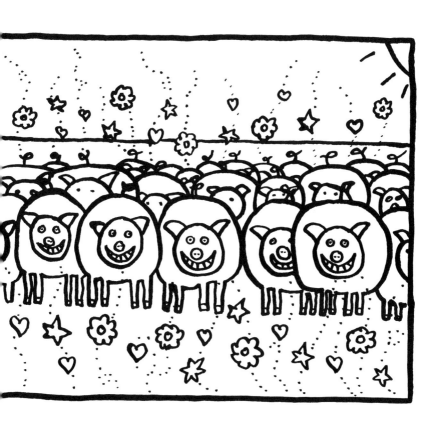

The SHEEP are
LAUGHING

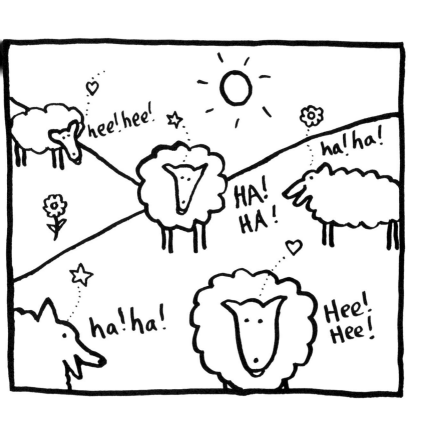

Even the CHICKENS
are beginning to
SMILE

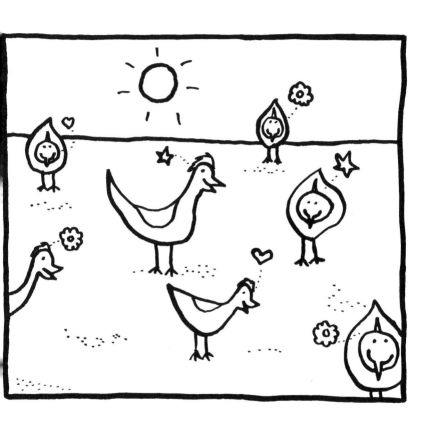

THE END